Tinnitus Triumph
"Conquering the Noise with Cognitive Behavioral Therapy"

Copyright © 2023 by Jills K. Kurian.
All rights reserved.

No part of this book may be reproduced, distributed, or transmitted in any form or by any means, including photocopying, recording, or other electronic or mechanical methods, without the prior written permission of the publisher, except in the case of brief quotations embodied in critical reviews and certain other non-commercial uses permitted by copyright law. For permission requests, write to the publisher, addressed "Attention: Permissions Coordinator," at the address below.

Publisher's Name: Jills K. Kurian
Publisher's Address: TRAGUS – The Ear Specialists, Regus, Admirals Park, Victory Way, Dartford, DA2 6QD.
Publisher's Email Address: support@tragusuk.com
Publisher's Website: https://tragusuk.com/

Table of Contents

Introduction 5
Chapter 1: Understanding Tinnitus and CBT 6
   1.1 What is Tinnitus? 6
   1.2 How CBT Works 6
   1.3 The Benefits of CBT for Tinnitus Sufferers 7
Chapter 2: Identifying Negative Thoughts 9
   2.1 Automatic Thoughts 9
   2.2 Intermediate Beliefs 9
   2.3 Core Beliefs 10
Chapter 3: Challenging Negative Thoughts 11
   3.1 Challenging Automatic Thoughts 11
   3.2 Challenging Intermediate Beliefs 12
   3.3 Challenging Core Beliefs 13
Chapter 4: Developing Your Own Negative Thought Challenge 14
   4.1 Identifying Your Personal Negative Thoughts 14
   4.2 Categorizing Your Thoughts Using the CBT Model 14

4.3 Creating Counterarguments and New Acceptable Thoughts 15

4.4 Practicing the Negative Thought Challenge 15

Chapter 5: Additional Support and Resources 17

5.1 Tinnitus Support Groups 17

5.2 Tinnitus Management Techniques 17

5.3 Mental Health Resources for Tinnitus Sufferers . 18

5.4 Further Reading and References 19

Conclusion 21

Summary 23

References 24

Tinnitus Support 25

Introduction

Tinnitus, the perception of ringing, buzzing, or hissing sounds in the absence of external stimuli, affects millions of people worldwide. For many, it's more than just a physical condition; it's a psychological burden that can lead to anxiety, depression, and other mental health challenges. The good news is that cognitive-behavioural therapy (CBT) offers a proven method for combating negative thoughts and improving quality of life.

This book aims to guide tinnitus sufferers through the process of challenging negative thoughts using CBT. By providing examples of common negative thoughts, categorizing them using the CBT model, and offering counterarguments and new acceptable thoughts, we aim to help readers train themselves to carry out the negative thought challenge independently.

Chapter 1:
Understanding Tinnitus and CBT

1.1 What is Tinnitus?

Tinnitus is a perception of noise or ringing in the ears or head when no external sound is present. It can manifest as various types of sounds, such as buzzing, hissing, or humming, and can range from mild to severe. Tinnitus affects millions of people around the world and can be caused by various factors, including hearing loss, exposure to loud noise, ear infections, or certain medications.

Although tinnitus is a common symptom, it is not a disease itself. It is often a symptom of an underlying condition, and its severity and impact on a person's life can vary significantly. For some, tinnitus may be a minor annoyance, while for others, it can lead to significant distress and negatively impact their quality of life.

1.2 How CBT Works

Cognitive-behavioral therapy (CBT) is a psychological treatment that aims to help individuals identify and change negative thought patterns, beliefs, and behaviors that contribute to emotional distress and life difficulties. It is based on the principle that our thoughts, emotions, and behaviors are interconnected, and by changing one aspect, we can influence the others.

CBT is a structured, time-limited, and goal-oriented approach that involves working with a therapist or using self-help materials to learn and practice new skills. In the context of tinnitus, CBT focuses on helping individuals recognize and challenge unhelpful thoughts and beliefs about their condition, learn relaxation techniques, and adopt healthy behaviors to improve their ability to cope with tinnitus.

1.3 The Benefits of CBT for Tinnitus Sufferers

CBT has been proven effective in helping individuals with tinnitus manage their symptoms and improve their overall well-being. Some of the benefits of CBT for tinnitus sufferers include:

Reducing the distress and emotional impact of tinnitus: CBT can help individuals reframe their thoughts about tinnitus, which in turn can lead to reduced anxiety, depression, and distress associated with the condition.

Enhancing coping skills and strategies: CBT equips individuals with practical tools and techniques to manage their tinnitus symptoms, such as relaxation exercises, sound therapy, and mindfulness practices.

Improving quality of life: By addressing negative thoughts and beliefs about tinnitus, individuals can develop a more balanced perspective, which can lead to an improved quality of life and greater enjoyment in daily activities.

Reducing the risk of long-term psychological issues: By learning to cope with tinnitus more effectively, individuals are less likely to develop chronic anxiety, depression, or other mental health problems related to their condition.

Overall, CBT is a valuable tool for tinnitus sufferers looking to manage their symptoms, improve their mental well-being, and lead a fulfilling life despite their condition.

Chapter 2: Identifying Negative Thoughts

In this chapter, we'll present ten common negative thoughts experienced by tinnitus sufferers. We'll categorize them using the CBT model, which divides negative thoughts into three types: automatic thoughts, intermediate beliefs, and core beliefs.

2.1 Automatic Thoughts

Automatic thoughts are spontaneous, involuntary thoughts that arise in response to a specific situation or trigger. They often have a negative or distorted tone, which can contribute to emotional distress.

Example 1: "This noise will never stop."
Example 2: "I can't concentrate on anything because of the ringing."
Example 3: "I'll never get a good night's sleep again."
Example 4: "No one understands what I'm going through."

2.2 Intermediate Beliefs

Intermediate beliefs are more general thoughts or assumptions that underlie automatic thoughts. They are often based on personal experiences, values, or attitudes and can serve as a bridge between automatic thoughts and core beliefs.

Example 5: "Tinnitus is ruining my life."
Example 6: "I'll never be able to enjoy social events again."
Example 7: "My career is at risk because of my tinnitus."
Example 8: "I can't handle the stress of dealing with this condition."

2.3 Core Beliefs

Core beliefs are deeply held beliefs about oneself, others, and the world that have developed over time, often during childhood. They are central to a person's identity and can significantly influence their thoughts, emotions, and behaviors.

Example 9: "I'm a failure because I can't cope with tinnitus."
Example 10: "I'm unlovable because of my condition."

By identifying and categorizing these negative thoughts, tinnitus sufferers can better understand the thought patterns that contribute to their distress and begin to challenge and replace them with more balanced, helpful thoughts. In the next chapter, we'll explore how to challenge these negative thoughts and create counterarguments and new acceptable thoughts for each example.

Chapter 3: Challenging Negative Thoughts

This chapter will provide guidance on how to challenge each of the negative thoughts presented in Chapter 2. We'll provide counterarguments and new acceptable thoughts for each example.

3.1 Challenging Automatic Thoughts

Counterargument 1: Tinnitus is often manageable, and many people learn to habituate to the noise.
New Acceptable Thought: "The noise may not stop completely, but I can learn to manage it and live a fulfilling life."

Counterargument 2: There are strategies to improve concentration despite tinnitus, such as using white noise or relaxation techniques.
New Acceptable Thought: "I may need to adapt my approach, but I can still concentrate on tasks and enjoy my hobbies."

Counterargument 3: Sleep can be improved with relaxation techniques, creating a sleep-friendly environment, and seeking professional help if needed.

New Acceptable Thought: "I can explore strategies to improve my sleep and manage tinnitus at night."

Counterargument 4: Many people experience tinnitus, and support is available from friends, family, and professionals who understand the challenges.
New Acceptable Thought: "I am not alone in my struggle, and I can seek understanding and support from others."

3.2 Challenging Intermediate Beliefs

Counterargument 5: Many people with tinnitus lead fulfilling lives by finding effective coping strategies and support.
New Acceptable Thought: "Tinnitus is challenging, but I can take steps to regain control and improve my quality of life."

Counterargument 6: Social events can still be enjoyed by adjusting expectations, using hearing protection, and seeking support from friends and family.
New Acceptable Thought: "I may need to adapt, but I can still participate in social events and enjoy the company of others."

Counterargument 7: Tinnitus may be a challenge, but it doesn't have to define your career. You can explore accommodations, adjustments, and support to maintain your work life.
New Acceptable Thought: "I can find ways to manage my tinnitus at work and continue to pursue my career goals."

Counterargument 8: Learning to cope with tinnitus takes time, and seeking support and using various strategies can help you manage stress more effectively.
New Acceptable Thought: "I can develop better stress management skills and build resilience to handle tinnitus-related challenges."

3.3 Challenging Core Beliefs

Counterargument 9: Coping with tinnitus is a journey, and seeking help is a sign of strength, not failure.
New Acceptable Thought: "I am strong for seeking help and trying to overcome my tinnitus-related challenges."

Counterargument 10: Tinnitus doesn't define your worth or lovability. You are deserving of love and support.
New Acceptable Thought: "I am lovable and deserving of love, regardless of my tinnitus."

By challenging negative thoughts and replacing them with more balanced and helpful perspectives, tinnitus sufferers can reduce their emotional distress, enhance their coping skills, and improve their overall quality of life.

Chapter 4: Developing Your Own Negative Thought Challenge

In this chapter, we'll guide you through the process of creating your personalized negative thought challenge, helping you address your unique tinnitus-related thoughts and beliefs.

4.1 Identifying Your Personal Negative Thoughts

Begin by listing the negative thoughts you have about your tinnitus. These might be similar to the examples provided in Chapter 2 or completely different. You can use a journal, a smartphone app, or a simple piece of paper to keep track of these thoughts as they arise throughout your day.

4.2 Categorizing Your Thoughts Using the CBT Model

Once you've compiled a list of your personal negative thoughts, categorize them using the CBT model into automatic thoughts, intermediate beliefs, and core beliefs. This categorization will help you better understand the nature of your thoughts and target them effectively.

4.3 Creating Counterarguments and New Acceptable Thoughts

For each negative thought you've identified, develop a counterargument that challenges the thought's validity or accuracy. Use evidence from your own life, research on tinnitus, and the examples provided in Chapter 3 as inspiration. Then, create a new acceptable thought that reflects a more balanced and helpful perspective.

4.4 Practicing the Negative Thought Challenge

Implementing the negative thought challenge takes practice and consistency. Use the following steps to make this process a habit:

Step 1. Notice when a negative thought arises in your mind.
Step 2. Recognize the thought's category (automatic, intermediate, or core belief).
Step 3. Remind yourself of the counterargument and new acceptable thought you've developed.
Step 4. Replace the negative thought with the new acceptable thought and refocus on your present moment or task.

Over time, practicing the negative thought challenge can help you change unhelpful thought patterns, reduce emotional distress, and improve your coping skills related to tinnitus.

Remember, developing and maintaining a positive mindset takes time and effort, so be patient with yourself and celebrate small victories along the way. By consistently practicing the negative thought challenge, you can gradually transform your thoughts, emotions, and behaviors, ultimately improving your quality of life despite tinnitus.

Chapter 5: Additional Support and Resources

In this chapter, we'll provide information on additional support and resources available to help you manage your tinnitus and maintain your mental well-being.

5.1 Tinnitus Support Groups

Support groups can be an invaluable resource for tinnitus sufferers, as they provide a safe space for individuals to share their experiences, learn from others, and find emotional support. Many support groups are available both in-person and online. Some places to find tinnitus support groups include:

- Local hospitals or clinics
- Tinnitus organizations, such as the American Tinnitus Association (ATA)
- Online forums and social media groups focused on tinnitus

5.2 Tinnitus Management Techniques

There are various techniques and approaches to help manage tinnitus symptoms. Some of these include:

- Sound therapy: Using white noise, nature sounds, or music to reduce the perception of tinnitus
- Hearing aids: For individuals with hearing loss, hearing aids may help alleviate tinnitus by improving hearing
- Tinnitus Retraining Therapy (TRT): A combination of sound therapy and counseling to help reduce tinnitus-related distress
- Mindfulness meditation: Practices that promote relaxation, stress reduction, and present-moment awareness
- Cognitive Behavioral Therapy (CBT): As discussed in this book, CBT can help challenge and change negative thought patterns related to tinnitus

5.3 Mental Health Resources for Tinnitus Sufferers

Taking care of your mental health is essential when dealing with tinnitus. Mental health resources for tinnitus sufferers include:

- Psychotherapy: Working with a mental health professional, such as a psychologist or counselor, can help you address the emotional impact of tinnitus
- Stress management: Learning techniques to manage stress, such as deep breathing exercises, progressive muscle relaxation, and visualization.
- Support from friends and family: Share your experiences with tinnitus and seek understanding and support from loved ones.

- Online resources: Websites, blogs, and forums dedicated to tinnitus and mental health can provide valuable information and support.

5.4 Further Reading and References

For additional information on tinnitus, its management, and the use of CBT for tinnitus, consider the following resources:

- American Tinnitus Association (ATA): https://www.ata.org/
- British Tinnitus Association (BTA): https://www.tinnitus.org.uk/
- Tragus - The Ear Specialists: https://www.tragusuk.com/
- Tinnitus: A Self-Management Guide for the Ringing in Your Ears by Jane L. Henry and Peter H. Wilson
- Cognitive Behavioral Therapy for Tinnitus by Eldré W. Beukes, Gerhard Andersson, and Vinaya Manchaiah
- Mindfulness for Tinnitus: A Practical Guide by Laurence McKenna and Liz Marks
- A New Harmony: Retraining Your Mind for Tinnitus Relief by Jills K Kurian

By utilizing the resources and support outlined in this chapter, you can better manage your tinnitus symptoms and improve your overall well-being. Remember, you are not alone in your journey, and there are many resources available to help you along the way.

Conclusion

Throughout this book, we have explored the challenges that tinnitus sufferers often face and how Cognitive Behavioral Therapy (CBT) can provide effective tools and strategies for managing the emotional impact of this condition. By understanding the nature of tinnitus and the power of CBT in challenging negative thoughts and beliefs, individuals can develop resilience and improve their quality of life despite their tinnitus symptoms.

We have examined the different types of negative thoughts that tinnitus sufferers commonly experience, along with practical guidance on how to challenge these thoughts using counterarguments and new acceptable thoughts. By applying these techniques, you can gradually transform your mindset and alleviate the emotional distress associated with tinnitus.

Furthermore, we have provided a step-by-step guide on developing your personalized negative thought challenge to help you address your unique tinnitus-related thoughts and beliefs. With consistent practice, you can learn to manage the impact of tinnitus on your mental and emotional well-being more effectively.

In addition to the CBT strategies covered in this book, we have highlighted various support groups, tinnitus management techniques, mental health resources, and further reading materials to assist you in your journey towards better tinnitus management. It is essential to remember that you are not alone in your struggle with tinnitus, and there is a wealth of resources and support available to help you.

As you continue to implement the techniques and strategies outlined in this book, be patient with yourself and celebrate your progress, no matter how small it may seem. Changing thought patterns and developing resilience takes time, effort, and commitment. Remember that setbacks are a normal part of the process and that it is essential to approach your journey with self-compassion and determination.

In conclusion, the journey towards better tinnitus management and improved mental well-being is an ongoing process. By using the principles of CBT and the practical guidance provided in this book, you can develop the skills and confidence to face your tinnitus-related challenges head-on. By harnessing the power of a positive mindset, seeking support, and utilizing the resources available, you can pave the way to a fulfilling life despite the presence of tinnitus.

Summary

Tinnitus can be a challenging condition to live with, but by utilizing CBT techniques to challenge negative thoughts, it's possible to improve your mental well-being and overall quality of life. This book has provided examples, counterarguments, and new acceptable thoughts to help guide you in your journey towards triumphing over tinnitus. Remember that seeking support from professionals, support groups, and loved ones is crucial in overcoming the challenges associated with tinnitus.

References

Cima, R. F. F., Maes, I. H., Joore, M. A., Scheyen, D. J. W. M., El Refaie, A., & Baguley, D. M. (2012). Specialised treatment based on cognitive behaviour therapy versus usual care for tinnitus: a randomised controlled trial. The Lancet, 379(9830), 1951-1959.

Henry, J. A., Stewart, B. J., & Griest, S. E. (2015). Tinnitus management: A comprehensive guide for the clinician. Plural Publishing.

McKenna, L., Marks, E. M., & Vogt, F. (2018). Cognitive behavioural therapy for tinnitus. Cochrane Database of Systematic Reviews, 1(1), CD012614.

Tyler, R. S. (Ed.). (2012). Tinnitus Treatment: Clinical Protocols. Thieme Medical Publishers.

Tinnitus Support

American Tinnitus Association: www.ata.org
British Tinnitus Association: www.tinnitus.org.uk
Tinnitus Hub: www.tinnitushub.com
Tinnitus Talk Support Forum: www.tinnitustalk.com

Note: This book is meant as a guide to assist tinnitus sufferers in understanding and challenging their negative thoughts. It is not intended to replace professional help or medical advice. If you're struggling with tinnitus, please consult a healthcare professional or a mental health expert with experience in tinnitus management.